D0297457

Spine Injuries

Gregory R. Houghton

Consultant and Honorary Lecturer
in Trauma and Orthopaedics
John Radcliffe Hospital and
Nuffield Orthopaedic Centre, Oxford, UK.

J.B. Lippincott Company ● Philadelphia
Gower Medical Publishing ● London ● New York

Distributed in USA and Canada by:

J.B. Lippincott Company
East Washington Square
Philadelphia, PA 19105
USA

Distributed in UK and Continental Europe by:

Harper & Row Ltd
Middlesex House
34-42 Cleveland Street
London W1P 5FB, UK

Distributed in Australia and New Zealand by:

Harper & Row (Australiasia) Pty Ltd
PO Box 226
Artarmon, NSW 2064
Australia

**Distributed in Philippines/Guam, Middle East,
Latin America and Africa by:**

Harper & Row International
10 East 53rd Street
New York, NY 10022
USA

**Distributed in Southeast Asia, Hong Kong,
India and Pakistan by:**

Harper & Row Publishers (Asia) Pte Ltd
37 Jalan Pemimpin 02-01
Singapore 2057

Distributed in Japan by:

Igaku Shoin Ltd
Tokyo International
PO Box 5063
Tokyo, Japan

British Library Cataloguing in Publication Data

Houghton, Gregory R
Spine injuries.
1. Spine & spinal cord. Injuries.
I. Title II. Series
617'482

ISBN: 397-44577-6 (Lippincott/Gower)

Project Editor: Gillian Lancaster
Design: Marie McNestry

Originated in Hong Kong by Imago Publishing Ltd
Printed in Hong Kong
Set in Sabon and Frutiger by Ampersand.

Gregory Houghton

The author was tragically killed in a road traffic accident and died on 18th September 1988. Greg. was a brilliant young man. He was a gifted orthopaedic surgeon and his particular interest was the spine. He had already received international recognition for his spinal research and it was quite clear to us all that over the next few years Greg., who was only just setting out on his career at the age of 43, was about to make a number of extremely important contributions over the next few years to our understanding of the spine. His untimely death has robbed the spinal world of a major contributor and those of us who knew him of a delightful friend. This book is an excellent example of the clear, incisive approach that Greg. brought to any subject that he tackled.

John Dove F.R.C.S.
Secretary, British Scoliosis Society   January 1989

CONTENTS

INTRODUCTION

With the development of modern imaging methods, particularly computerized tomography, there is a better understanding of spinal injuries, both from the point of view of injury mechanisms and planning treatment. Injuries to the spinal column continue to account for a high proportion of long-term morbidity following trauma. Despite changes in traffic laws, safer mining practices and better protection for the sportsman, there has not been a significant drop in the overall incidence of spinal injury.

Traditionally, the majority of spinal injuries have been treated conservatively by bedrest and support until the fracture has healed, when mobilization is begun. More recently, a more interventionist approach has been advocated, with the aims of fracture reduction, spinal cord decompression, and surgical stabilization. Such an approach is aimed at early rehabilitation, reduction of post-injury pain, and allowing the best conditions for neurological recovery. As with long bone trauma, there are indications for both operative and conservative management.

By illustrating the principles of spinal injuries, as well as the more common injury patterns and their management, it is hoped that this book will lead to a clear understanding of spinal trauma, particularly by those who manage the patients soon after injury.

Inevitably some patients sustain irrecoverable neurological damage. It is hoped that with proper early care, the number of such patients in this group might be reduced.

FIRST AID CARE

Although the maximum injury to the spine is likely to be caused at the moment of impact, poor handling of the patient, particularly if he is unconscious, may cause further damage. The following rules must be adhered to:

- Assume a spinal injury is present.
- Examine the entire patient for external signs of injury.
- When moving the patient, apply light manual traction to the neck, and move the neck and torso as a unit, avoiding angulation or torsion (Fig.1).

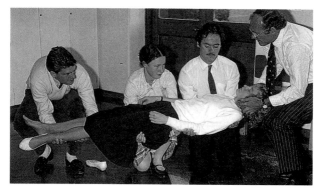

Fig.1 Moving the patient.

STABLE OR UNSTABLE?

The stable spine is safe and although damage to bones and ligaments may have occurred, such damage is not sufficient for subsequent movements of the spine to cause further displacement with risk to neurological structures.

The spine may be considered to consist of three columns (Fig.2). If only one column is damaged, the spine is stable, but if two or three columns are involved, the spine is, by definition, unstable.

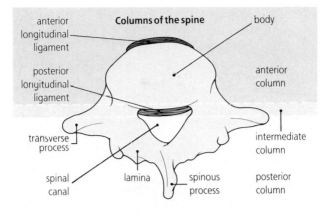

Fig.2 Columns of the spine shown on a cross-section (superior aspect) of the fifth lumbar vertebra. The anterior column consists of most of the vertebral body, as well as the anterior longitudinal ligament. The intermediate column includes the posterior part of the vertebral body, together with the closely applied posterior longitudinal ligament. The posterior column accounts for the remaining vertebral elements, including the posterior ligaments.

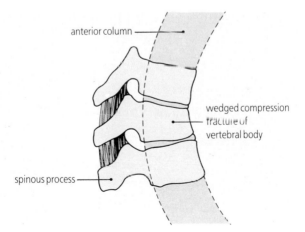

Fig.3 In a wedge compression fracture, only the anterior column is involved, as shown in this longitudinal section through the lower thoracic vertebrae. There is no incursion by the fracture into the spinal canal indicated by the maintenance of the posterior body height. The posterior structures are undamaged.

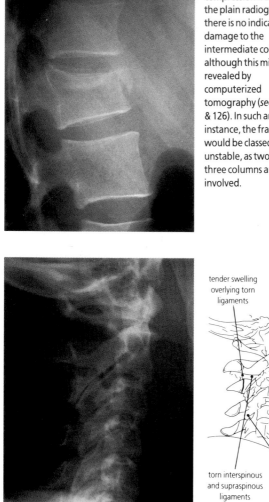

Fig.4 Stable compression fracture. On the plain radiograph there is no indication of damage to the intermediate column, although this might be revealed by computerized tomography (see Figs 125 & 126). In such an instance, the fracture would be classed as unstable, as two of the three columns are involved.

tender swelling overlying torn ligaments

torn interspinous and supraspinous ligaments

intact ligaments

Fig.5 Disruption of the posterior interspinous and supraspinous ligaments (right) is a disruption of the posterior column only and therefore stable. The radiograph (left) shows no bony injury, but the injury is assumed because of the increased distance between C3 and C4 spinous processes. Clinically, the increased interspinous distance can be appreciated as well as a tender swelling.

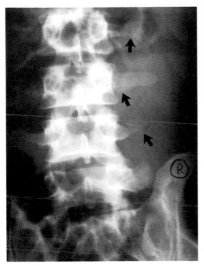

Fig.6 Fractures of the transverse processes (arrows) involve the posterior spinal column only. The spinal canal is not affected and this is a stable injury.

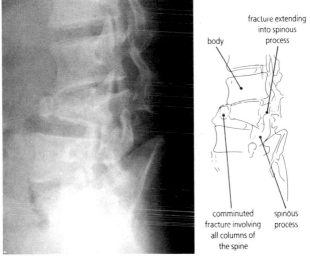

fracture extending into spinous process

body

comminuted fracture involving all columns of the spine

spinous process

Fig.7 Comminuted fracture involving disruption of the vertebral body and spinous process. Severe ligamentous and intervertebral disc disruption is an inevitable component of such an injury. Special radiographic views including computerized tomography are needed for accurate evaluation of such an injury.

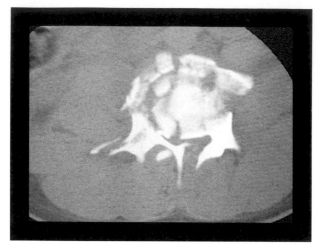

Fig.8 Computerized tomography of an unstable fracture. There is gross comminution of the vertebral body, pedicles and laminae; the spine is grossly unstable, as all three columns of the spine are involved.

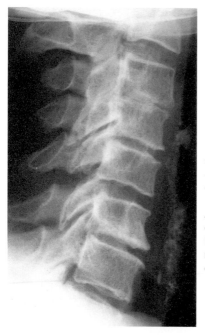

Fig.9 Occasionally, a spine may be unstable with ligamentous injury only. Here, there is clear separation of C5 and C6 vertebrae, both between the vertebral bodies anteriorly and the spinous processes and facet joints posteriorly (arrowed). Moderate soft tissue swelling is present anteriorly and this has displaced the calcified larynx forwards. Although this patient is elderly, unstable, purely ligamentous injuries are more common in children.

NEUROLOGICAL DAMAGE

The importance of spinal injuries depends upon whether or not there is neurological damage sustained at the time of injury, and the level of injury.

Types of lesion:
- Acute cord crush. This usually results in a complete and irreversible neurological lesion.
- Cord compression by bone or disc. The lesion may cause a partial or total neurological injury.
- Vascular cord damage. This can occur without fracture, particularly in children and the elderly with cervical spondylosis. The level of injury may extend following vessel thrombosis.

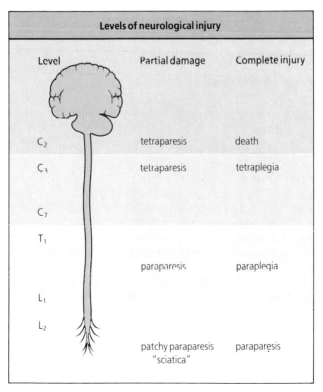

Fig.10 Levels of neurological injury.

UPPER CERVICAL INJURIES

A clear history of injury to the neck with resulting pain and deformity will present no difficulty in diagnosis of neck injury after relevant radiographs have been carried out. Often a clear history is not available and so a high index of suspicion should lead the doctor to assume that a spine injury is present unless it is positively excluded. The cervical spine should be radiographed in the following circumstances:

- Neck pain following trauma.
- With a head injury in the unconscious patient.
- If the patient is conscious, the neck should be radiographed, particulary if there is external evidence of bone injury to the face (Fig.11) or to the skull vault (Fig.12).
- Torticollis following injury (Fig.13).
- Abrasions or bruising about the neck (Fig.14).
- Paralysis following injury.

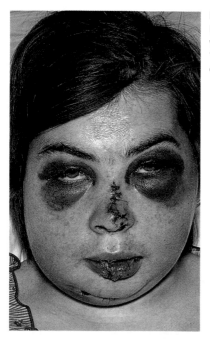

Fig.11 Patient with a Le Fort type II facial fracture, who sustained a 'whiplash' injury to the cervical spine (*see* Fig.62).

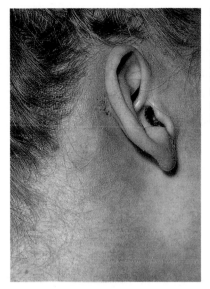

Fig.12 Bruising of the occipital region with blood in the external auditory meatus, indicating a base of skull fracture. This patient sustained an upper cervical spine ligamentous injury.

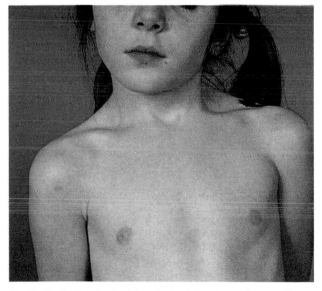

Fig.13 Torticollis following injury. Such a deformity may be caused by spinal column fracture or dislocation or more commonly with muscle spasm accompanying soft tissue injury.

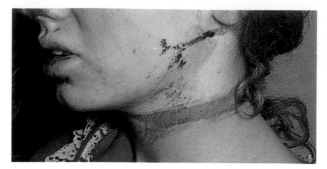

Fig.14 Abrasions around the neck.

ATLANTOAXIAL INJURIES

These are potentially the most serious of spinal injuries, as complete cord damage at C1 or C2 results in diaphragmatic paralysis (C3, C4, C5) and death.

Congenital Anomalies

These are common throughout the axial skeleton and occur in approximately 15% of the population. Anomalies occur most frequently at the upper and lower ends of the spine. Fig.16 shows asymmetric development of the atlantoaxial joints. Such a radiograph may be erroneously interpreted as the post-traumatic deformity. Congenital spinal anomalies are more susceptible to injury than the normally developed spine.

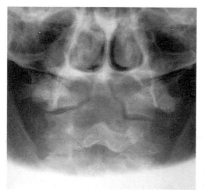

Fig.15 Occipitoatlantic subluxation. This is a rare anomaly, recognized after a rugby injury and resulting in chronic neck pain. There is poor development of the occipital condyles, predisposing to subluxation with minimal injury. As with many spinal conditions, only tomography would reveal the full extent of the lesion.

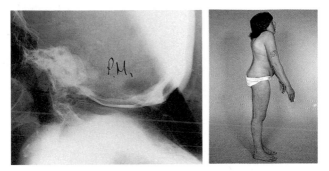

Fig.16 The Klippel – Feil syndrome is a common cervical spine anomaly (left) with congenital vertebral fusion leading to vulnerability of any uninvolved mobile segments, particularly at the atlantoaxial region. (*See also* Fig.24.) The clinical appearance (right) is typical and shows marked shortening of the neck, together with congenital shoulder elevation.

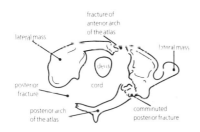

fracture of anterior arch of the atlas
lateral mass
lateral mass
dens
posterior fracture
cord
posterior arch of the atlas
comminuted posterior fracture

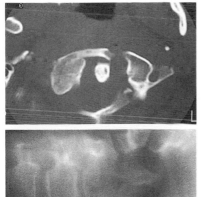

Fig.17 A burst fracture of the atlas. This 'Jefferson' fracture is caused by vertical compression, such as diving into a shallow pool. The orientation of the occipital condyles forces the lateral masses of the atlas apart, so that the ring of the atlas bursts centrifugally, as shown by the gaps between the fracture fragments. The cord is thus often spared. A computerized tomograph of the atlas shows the increased dimensions of the vertebral canal owing to separation of the fracture fragments. The anteroposterior view (lower) shows separation of the lateral masses of the atlas.

Odontoid Fractures

Odontoid fractures are usually caused by high-velocity injuries and are often fatal. The commonest type (type II) renders the spine unstable. The spine must be stabilized either by external support or surgery, as minimal trauma may displace the fracture further and result in sudden death.

Classification of odontoid fractures

- *Type I.* The least common variety, with an apical fracture of the dens caused by avulsion by the apical ligament. Most of the dens is intact and the spine is stable. Long-term problems do not occur.
- *Type II.* The commonest odontoid fracture occurs though the base of the dens. These fractures are unstable. As the majority of the blood supply passes to the dens from the body of the axis, both fracture non-union and avascular necrosis are common. Atlantoaxial fusion is therefore frequently indicated.
- *Type III.* These fractures involve the well vascularized cancellous bone of the body of the axis and therefore usually unite after a period of external immobilization.

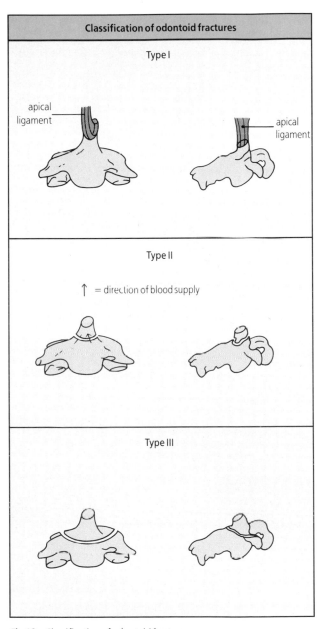

Fig.18 Classification of odontoid fractures.

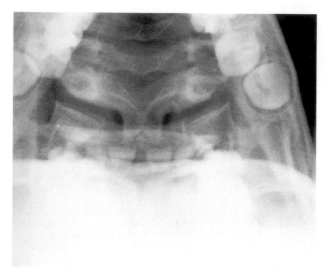

Fig.19 Type I. Apical fracture is best visualized as an open mouth view of the dens. The fracture had united after 6 weeks of support in a collar without complication.

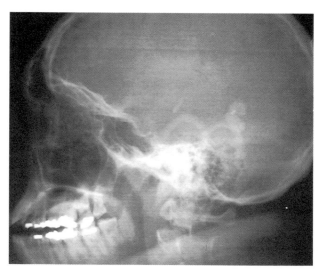

Fig.20 A displaced type II fracture was noted on the lateral view of a series of skull radiographs in a patient injured in a car accident. Cervical spine injury should be suspected in all unconscious patients.

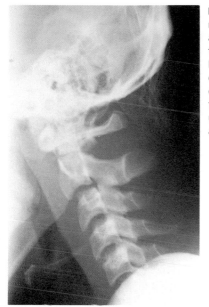

Fig.21 An accurate reduction has been achieved with skull traction using tongs (*see* Fig.52). Despite this degree of reduction, over one third of type II fractures progress to non-union and require atlantoaxial fusion.

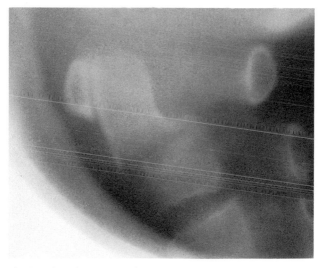

Fig.22 A lateral tomogram of a type III basal odontoid fracture with little displacement. Union is to be anticipated after 6 – 12 weeks with a firm collar.

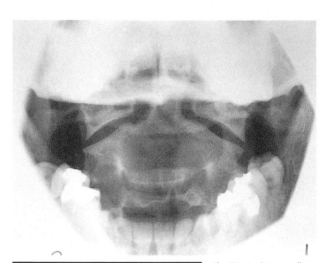

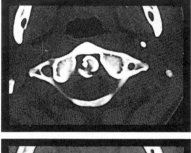

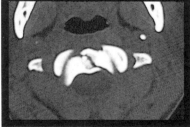

Fig.23 An intermediate type fracture between types II and III. The anteroposterior open mouth view (upper) shows an oblique fracture through the dens and the body of the axis. A CT scan (middle) confirms a vertical split in the dens, which is therefore less substantial than normal but functionally intact. The fracture is thus stable. A CT scan through the body of the axis (lower) shows the fracture through cancellous bone. The expected union occurred in 8 weeks with support in a collar.

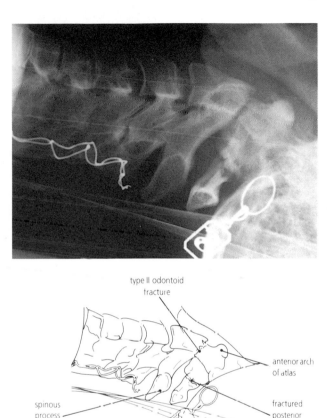

Fig.24 As with the Klippel – Feil syndrome (Fig. 16) this patient had a long cervical spine fusion (C3 to C7) following previous trauma (upper). The upper mobile segments are thus vulnerable and a mild blow to the head was complicated by a Jefferson burst fracture of the atlas and a type II odontoid fracture (lower).

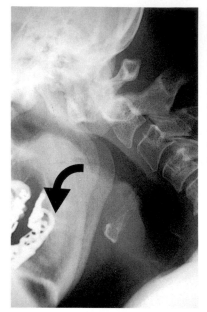

Fig. 25 Dislocation of the atlantoaxial joint is a rare injury unless the transverse ligament of the atlas is weakened by an inflammatory process, such as rheumatoid arthritis. This radiograph, taken in flexion, shows the degree of separation of the anterior arch of the atlas from the odontoid peg in a patient with rheumatoid arthritis.

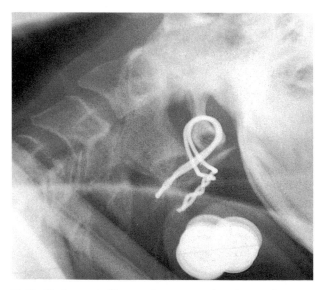

Fig. 26 The ligament will not repair spontaneously and a posterior atlantoaxial fusion with support from a transfixion wire is indicated.

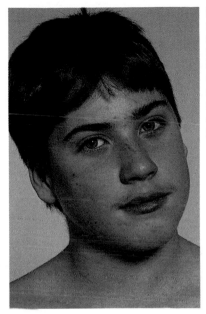

Fig.27 Atlantoaxial rotatory subluxation is an often undiagnosed injury to the atlantoaxial ligaments. It usually occurs in children and results in a characteristic tilt of the head – the so-called 'cock robin' position.

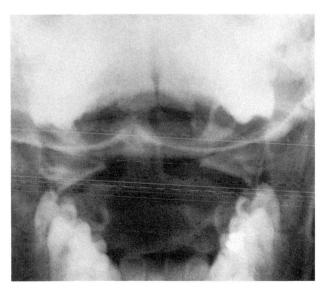

Fig.28 A transoral radiograph is diagnostic in atlantoaxial subluxation and shows eccentricity of the dens between the lateral masses of the atlas.

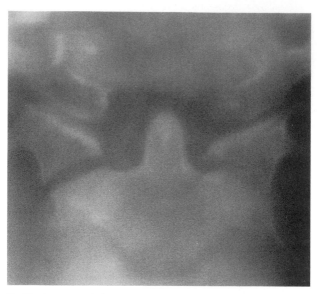

Fig.29 A tomograph shows unilateral facet subluxation.

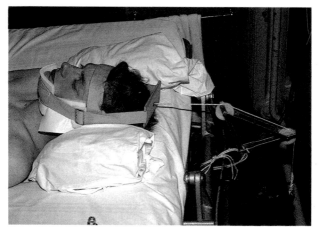

Fig.30 The injury settles if treated early with halter traction followed by support in an orthosis until symptoms resolve.

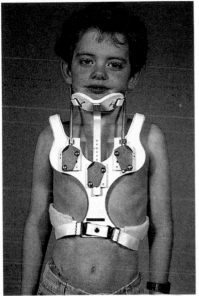

Fig.31 An occipito-mentothoracic orthosis used to support the cervical spine in conditions such as atlantoaxial rotatory subluxation.

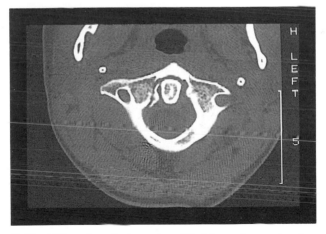

Fig.32 A CT scan shows the true nature of the injury – a bony avulsion by the insertion of the transverse ligament of the lateral mass.

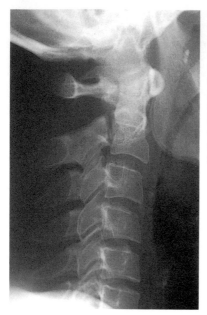

Fig.33 Radiograph of a hangman's fracture sustained during a car accident. The injury is a traumatic spondylolisthesis of the pedicles of the axis resulting in subluxation between C2 and C3. There was no neurological deficit sustained in this unstable injury.

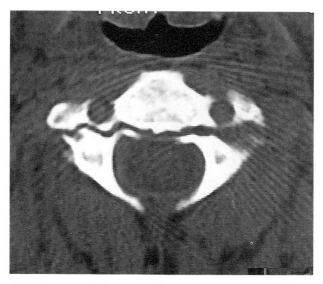

Fig.34 A computerized tomogram shows minimal displacement of the fracture.

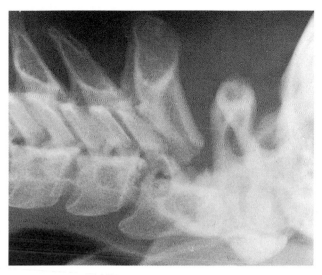

Fig.35 A markedly displaced hangman's fracture with gross dislocation between C2 and C3. Such a degree of displacement is usually fatal because of respiratory paralysis.

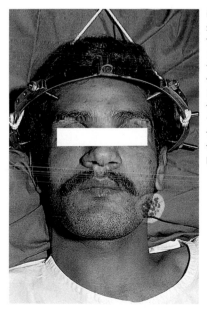

Fig.36 Unstable cervical spine injuries are best treated initially in halo traction with four pins fixed to the outer table of the skull. In most instances this is superior to skull traction with 'tongs' which are fixed by two pins only, and therefore less stable (see Fig.52).

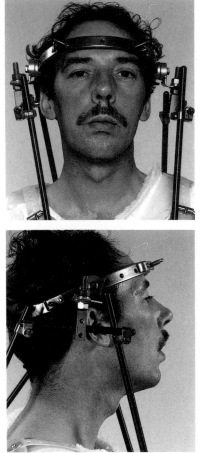

Fig.37 A halo can be secured to a body jacket which permits the patient to be mobilized early whilst an unstable cervical injury is rigidly held.

THE MID AND LOWER CERVICAL SPINE

The mid-cervical spine is well evaluated radiographically by anteroposterior, lateral, and forty-five degree supine oblique films (to visualize the facet joints and root canals). The cervicothoracic junction, however, is often difficult to image, particularly in 'short-necked', obese men. If cervical spine injury is suspected, it is essential to visualize the cervicothoracic junction, using either a traction view or a 'swimmer's' view.

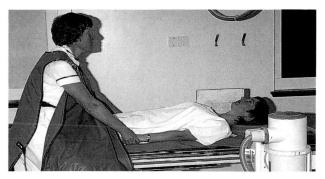

Fig.38 Traction views of the cervical spine are taken with the head steadied and the shoulders held down. This manoeuvre is often required to visualize the cervicothoracic junction.

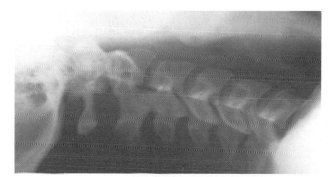

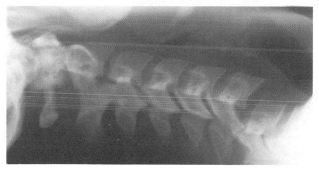

Fig.39 This lateral radiograph of the cervical spine (upper) shows only six cervical vertebrae, all of which are uninjured. A traction view of the same patient (lower) shows the entire C7 vertebra, and an obvious major fracture dislocation at the C6/C7 level.

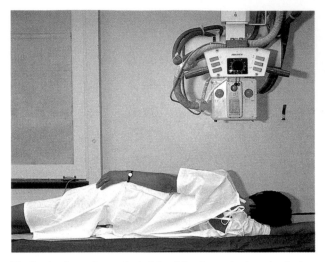

Fig.40 An alternative method of visualizing the cervicothoracic spine is the 'swimmer's' view, in which the shoulders are so positioned that they do not obscure the C7/T1 region.

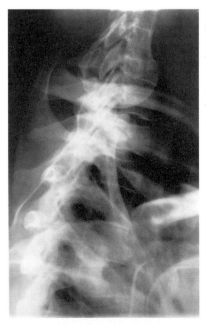

Fig.41 A radiograph of a swimmer's view of the cervicothoracic junction. Although the spine can be delineated, confusion may occur owing to overlying bone and soft tissue shadows.

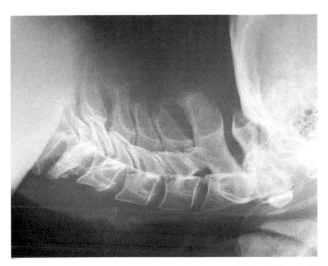

Fig.42 A burst fracture of C6 caused by a fall from a height onto the skull vertex. There is little intrusion by bone of the spinal canal and there was no cord damage. The fracture is stable and should be treated in a firm collar.

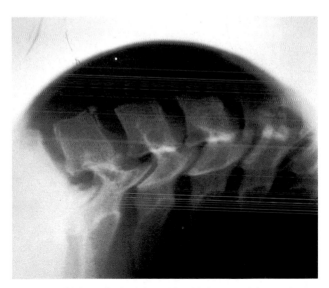

Fig.43 A stable hyperflexion injury with a chip fracture of the anterior margin of the superior bone plate of C6. This injury is treated symptomatically with a collar which holds the neck in extension.

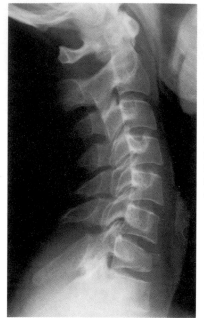

Fig.44 A more severe hyperflexion injury with a wedge compression fracture of the body of C7. Separation of the spinous processes of C6 and C7 indicate damage to the supraspinous and interspinous ligaments. The facet joints are undamaged and as the spine is stable in extension, it may be supported in a cervicothoracic support.

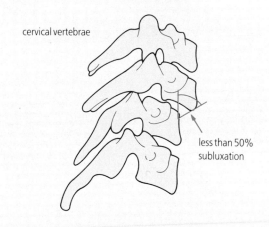

cervical vertebrae

less than 50% subluxation

Fig.45 Unifacet dislocation of the cervical spine is a flexion/rotation injury and usually escapes neurological complication. There is less than 50% subluxation between adjacent bodies, as seen on a lateral radiograph.

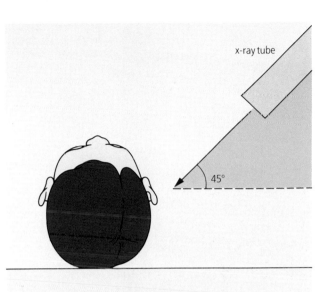

Fig.16 A 45° supine oblique radiograph identifies the side of facet dislocation. This is necessary if manipulation is to be carried out.

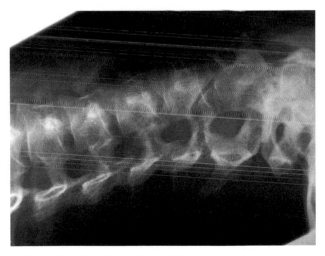

Fig.47 A 45° supine oblique radiograph showing normal nerve root foraminae and posterior facet joints. No facet dislocation is evident.

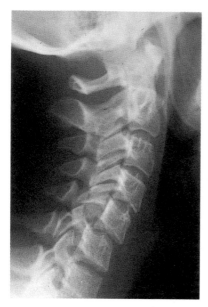

Fig.48 This unifacet dislocation was treated by gradual skull traction until reduction occurred, when the neck was supported in a cervicothoracic support.

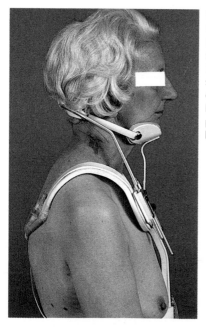

Fig.49 A cervicothoracic orthosis, suitable for support of a painful, but stable, cervical spine injury. This patient had suffered a unifacet dislocation, which had been reduced one week previously. Extensive neck bruising is present.

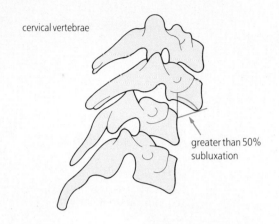

cervical vertebrae

greater than 50%
subluxation

Fig.50 Bilateral facet dislocation usually results in a complete cord injury, and is diagnosed on a lateral film as a greater than 50% subluxation between adjacent cervical spine bodies.

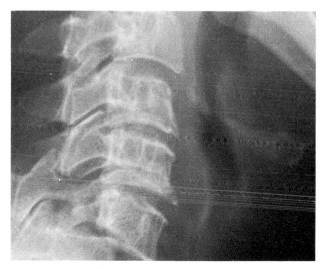

Fig.51 C6 – C7 bilateral facet dislocation with complete tetraplegia. The facets are locked so that hyperextension will not reduce the dislocation. Sustained heavy skull traction usually causes separation of the locked facets and subsequent reduction.

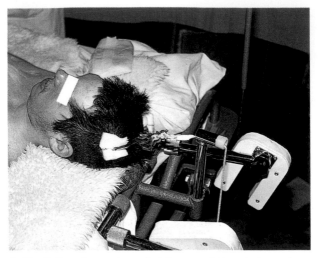

Fig.52 Skull traction may be applied via tongs, which can be inserted under local anaesthesia. Up to 20kg of traction may be applied by this means, and this is usually enough to reduce bilateral facet dislocation. Tong traction has been largely superceded by halo traction, which can be fitted to a body jacket (see Figs 36 and 37).

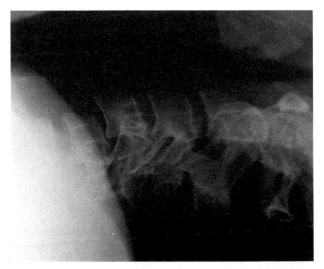

Fig.53 A 50% fracture dislocation between C4 and C5 with complete paraplegia and sparing of the diaphragm.

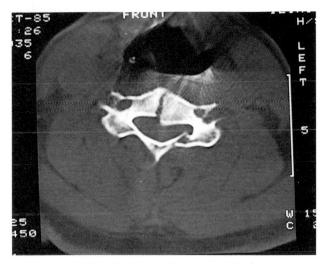

Fig.54 A CT scan shows the fracture to be more complex than appears on plain films, with a sagittal fracture through the body and posterior arch.

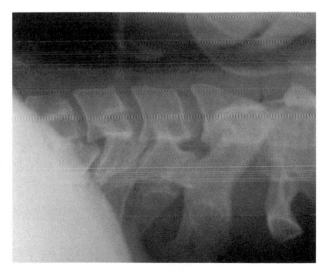

Fig.55 Fracture reduction was achieved within 30 minutes using 13.6kg of traction under sedation. There was no neurological recovery.

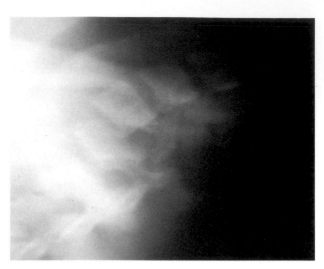

Fig.56 Tomograph of a patient with C6/C7 dislocation due to unilateral facet fracture. The injury was complicated by Brown – Sequard syndrome (*see* Fig. 97).

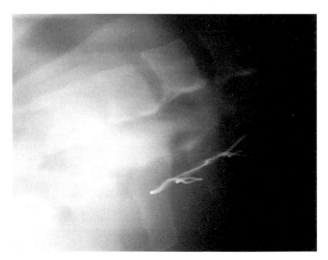

Fig.57 Traction did not result in reduction, so open reduction and fusion with an interspinous wire and autogenous bone graft was carried out. The patient made a complete neurological recovery. This case illustrates the clinical axiom that partial lesions often recover and complete lesions rarely do, irrespective of the extent of vertebral trauma.

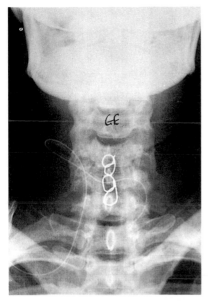

Fig.58 Anteroposterior view showing stabilization of the dislocation with interspinous wiring.

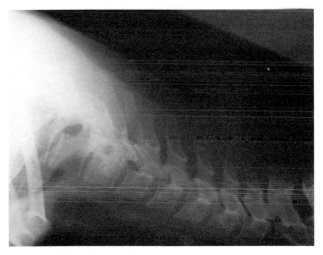

Fig.59 Fracture of the spinous process of C7. This is known as the clay shovellers' fracture, which affects either C7 or T1, or rarely both vertebrae. It is an avulsion injury caused by violent contraction of the muscles attached to the spinous processes, especially the trapezius, during heavy manual activities.

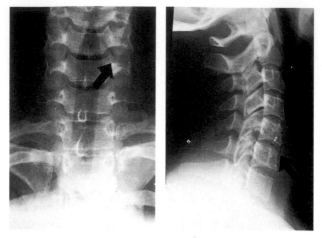

Fig.60 Isolated fracture of the lamina caused by a hyperextension injury. Such a fracture does not result in cord damage but may sometimes be seen in whiplash injuries. The fracture readily unites in a collar.

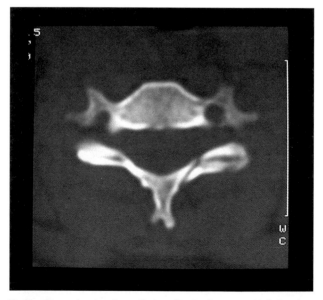

Fig.61 CT scan showing the undisplaced lamina fracture, with little soft tissue involvement. Clinically, this presents with minor muscle spasm only and no external signs of injury.

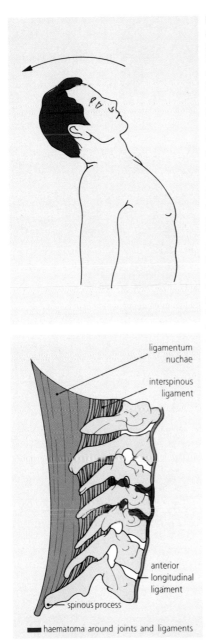

Fig.62 Whiplash injury is a very common and poorly understood neck injury caused by hyper-extension of the neck (upper), such as occurs when a car is struck from behind. The head is thrust backwards, compressing the posterior elements and stretching the anterior ligaments. This is followed by a rebound hyperflexion of the neck with stretching of the posterior ligaments. Tearing of the ligaments results (lower), but bony injury is unusual. As well as neck pain, seemingly unrelated symptoms, such as vertigo, blurred vision, headaches and depression, may occur, although complete recovery with prolonged collar wear is the usual outcome.

ligamentum nuchae

interspinous ligament

anterior longitudinal ligament

spinous process

haematoma around joints and ligaments

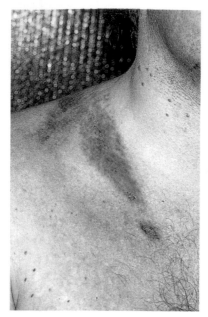

Fig.63 Safety belt restraint marks should alert the clinician to the possibility of injury at the cervicothoracic junction, where the neck is very flexible above the rigidly restrained thorax. Such spinal injuries are often accompanied by rib or clavicle fractures and brachial plexus or great vessel injury.

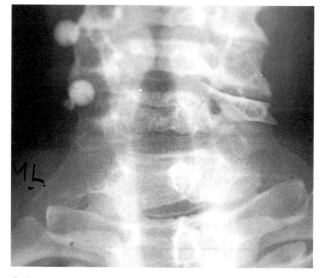

Fig.64 Fracture of the lateral mass of C7 with C7 nerve root neuropraxia in a restrained car driver. A complete recovery occurred.

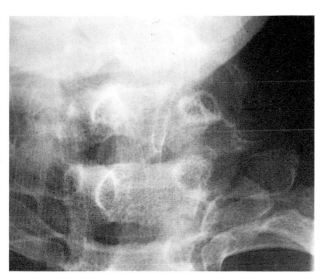

Fig.65 Fracture of the transverse process of the first thoracic vertebra in a restrained car passenger. Damage to the stellate ganglia occurred, resulting in Horner's syndrome.

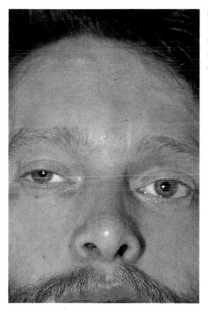

Fig.66 A patient with Horner's syndrome showing pin-point pupil, ptosis and enophthalmos of the right eye.

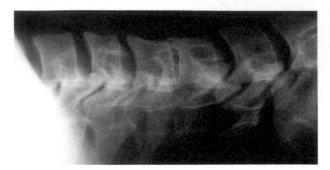

Fig.67 Coexistant congenital abnormalities seen on radiographs may be confusing following spinal trauma. In this case a fusion of C4 and C5 was suspected initially as a site of trauma following a head injury sustained in a road traffic accident.

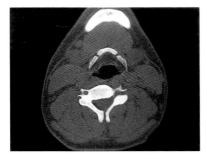

Fig.68 The congenital abnormality in this case is confirmed on CT scanning when a spina bifida occulta of C4 is demonstrated.

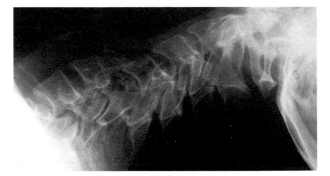

Fig.69 Diseased bone is more vulnerable to injury. This patient fell, sustaining a fracture dislocation through a metastasis of C5, with resulting tetraplegia.

THE THORACIC SPINE

Unlike the cervical or lumbar spine, the thoracic spine is relatively immobile and is protected from injury by the rib cage (Fig.70). Considerable force is therefore required to damage the thoracic spine, and fractures of the ribs or sternum and visceral injury to the heart, lungs, spleen or liver commonly accompany thoracic spine fracture.

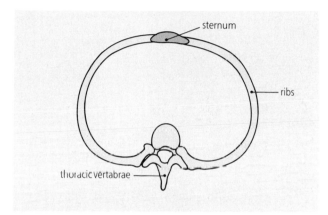

Fig.70 Transverse section through the thorax showing the thoracic spine protected by the rib cage.

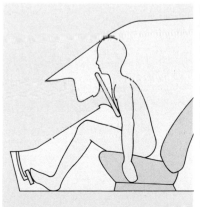

Fig.71 The commonest cause of fracture is a high-velocity accident, such as a road traffic accident. The chest of the victim either strikes the steering wheel or is acutely flexed across a safety belt. Mid thoracic fracture with a fractured sternum is a common injury complex.

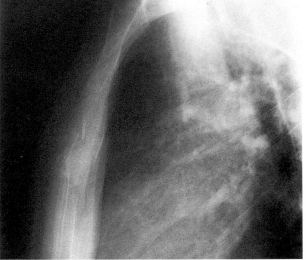

Fig.72 Fracture of the sternum. A radiograph such as this should alert the clinician to examine the thoracic viscera as well as the thoracic spine, where flexion injuries commonly occur (*see* Fig.80).

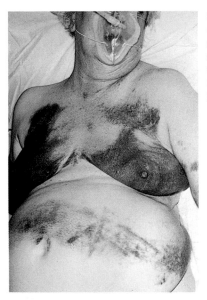

Fig.73 Extensive contusion caused by a seat belt. This patient suffered extensive chest wall injuries, as well as a ruptured spleen and a burst fracture of T7.

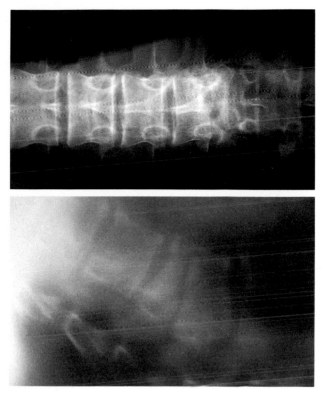

Fig.74 Fracture dislocation of T7. This view (upper) shows malalignment of spinous processes and pedicles, as well as loss of disc space and paravertebral haematoma. The lateral view (lower) shows the extent of the burst fracture and subluxation at T7. The patient suffered a partial paraplegia.

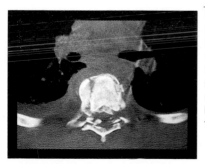

Fig.75 A CT scan of the same injury shows the true extent of the injury, with fractures involving all three columns of the spine. The spinal canal is markedly compromized by intrusion of fracture fragments.

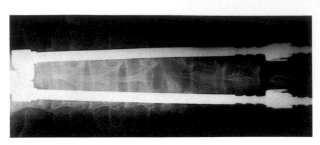

Fig.76 Treatment with double Harrington distraction rods, which both stabilize the spine and decompress the spinal canal.

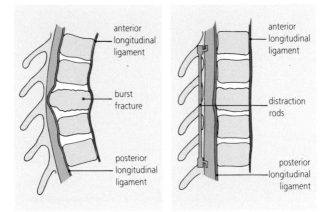

Fig.77 Distraction rod treatment for decompression of the spinal canal. The posterior longitudinal ligament (behind the vertebral bodies) is rarely ruptured in burst fractures (left), and distraction causes tension in the ligaments, which push retropulsed bone fragments back towards the vertebral body (right).

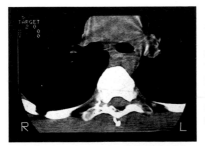

Fig.78 A CT scan taken after removal of the rods (one year after injury) shows reconstitution of the spinal canal. The partial paraplegia recovered with no residual neurological deficit.

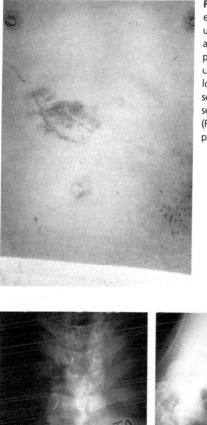

Fig.79 Careful examination of the torso usually reveals bruising if a thoracic injury is present, in this case caused by the high localized forces from a seat belt. The resulting severe spinal injury (Fig.80) caused complete paraplegia.

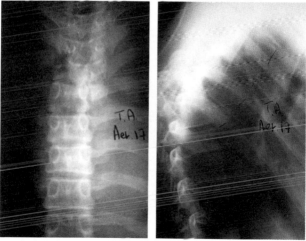

Fig.80 AP radiograph (left) showing gross fracture dislocation at the T5/T6 level. Such a 50% degree of subluxation invariably causes total paraplegia as the cord occupies most of the spinal canal in the thoracic region. The lateral radiograph (right) shows a 50° kyphos caused by a 50% subluxation in the sagittal plane, as well as wedging of the body of T5.

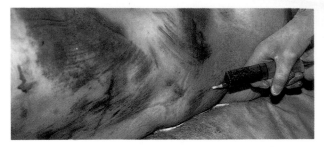

Fig.81 Diffuse extensive soft tissue injury of the torso, as in this victim of a road traffic accident, is less likely to cause a severe spinal injury. Aspiration of a superficial haematoma is shown.

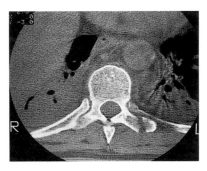

Fig.82 A CT scan of the same patient shows a fractured transverse process. The cord is not under threat, the fracture is stable, and no treatment is indicated.

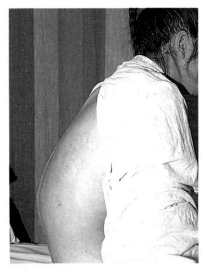

Fig.83 Spinal deformity in a schizophrenic woman who jumped from a bridge. The photograph was taken 4 days after injury, and the deformity is clearly stable, and, in this case, apparently painless.

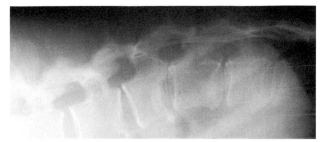

Fig.84 A radiograph of the previous patient shows multiple compression fractures involving only the anterior column of the spine, which is therefore stable.

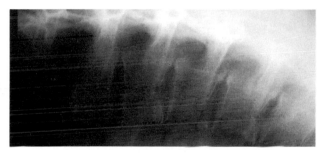

Fig.85 Multiple compression fractures in the spine of a 36-year-old man, who complained of thoracic back pain following an epileptic fit. The fractures were caused, not by a fall from a height, but by the intense muscle contractions sustained during the fit.

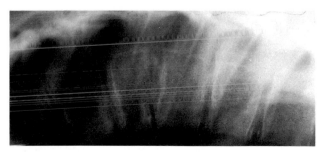

Fig.86 Scheuermann's disease of the thoracic spine, which may mimic compression fractures. The condition is most common in adolescent males and is manifest by multiple vertebral end plate irregularities, most commonly in the anterior parts of adjacent vertebral bodies at the thoracolumbar junction.

Pathological Fractures

The thoracic spine is the commonest site for pathological fractures. Generalized disease of bone may cause multiple wedge compression fractures or burst fractures. The bone is weakened by disease and only minimal force is needed for fracture to occur.

General causes of pathological fracture	
hereditary	osteogenesis imperfecta osteochondrodystrophy
acquired	osteoporosis osteomalacia & rickets osteodystrophy steroid therapy multiple myeloma leukaemia

Fig.87 General causes of pathological fracture.

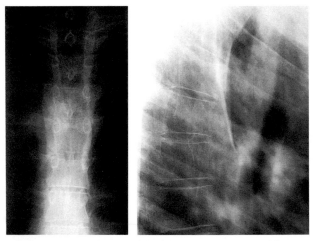

Fig.88 Compression fracture of the thoracic spine in a 68-year-old woman suffering from post-menopausal osteoporosis. Such fractures are painful but never cause spinal cord compression.

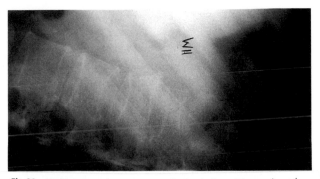

Fig.89 Multiple burst fractures caused by implosion of the weakened vertebral bodies by the discs. In this instance, the pathological process was osteomalacia following chronic kidney disease.

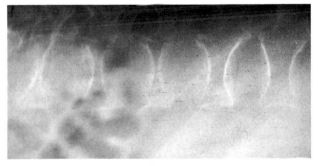

Fig.90 Multiple vertebral collapse in a child with severe osteogenesis imperfecta. The discs occupy much more of the anterior spinal column than the fragile vertebral bodies.

Tumours metastasising to bone		
1 breast	5 kidney	
2 bronchus	6 bowel	
3 prostate	7 lymphoma	
4 thyroid		

Fig.91 Tumours metastasizing to bone. Any tumour may cause bone metastases, but these are the commonest sources in order of frequency. Primary bone tumours are very rare.

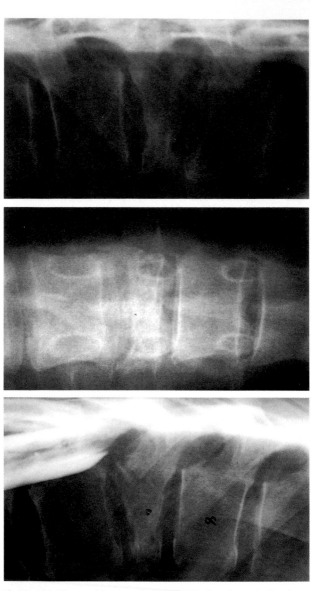

Fig.92 This 46-year-old woman slipped and developed paraplegia. The lateral radiograph (upper) shows collapse of the vertebral body. An AP radiograph (middle) showed the pedicles to be uninvolved. A myelogram (lower) showed a complete block caused by interior compression.

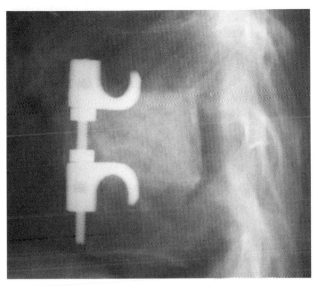

Fig.93 Anterior decompression and reconstruction with a distraction rod and bone cement was carried out, with complete recovery of the neurological lesion. The diagnosis was malignant lymphoma.

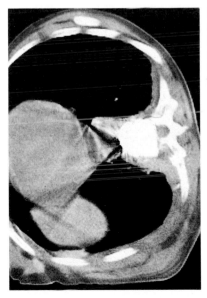

Fig.94 A CT scan showing a capacious spinal canal and replacement of the vertebral body by a block of methyl methacrylate.

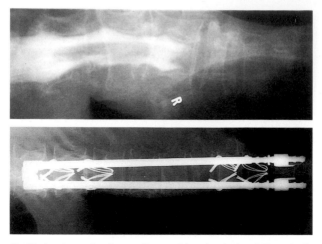

Fig.95 In advanced malignant disease of the spine the instability caused by bone destruction results in progressive paraplegia. In such cases, extensive anterior compression is unrealistic. The myelogram (upper) shows the extent of cord compression. The spine is decompressed by extensive laminectomy and stabilized with Harrington rods and sublaminar wires (lower) to prevent further neurological deterioration.

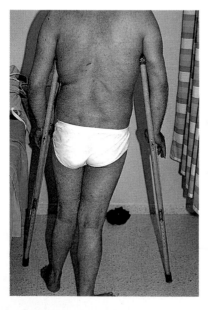

Fig.96 Open spinal injuries are very rare but stabbings to the thoracic region are becoming more common. A thin blade may be insinuated between the thoracic laminae and cause cord damage. This man has a 2cm entry wound and a hemicord lesion at T9, resulting in the Brown–Sequard syndrome.

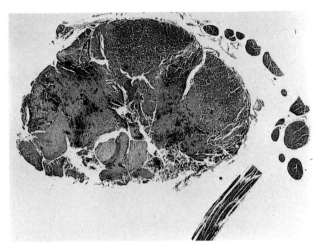

Fig.97 Transverse section of the spinal cord showing destruction of half the cord with (ipsilateral) hemiparesis and contralateral loss of pain and temperature sensation (Brown–Sequard syndrome).

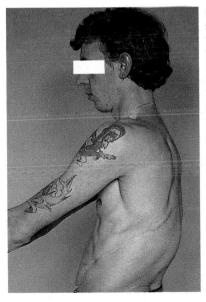

Fig.98 Without stabilization, spinal fractures, particularly in the thoracic region, may result in a painful kyphosis. Together with a thoracic fracture, this patient suffered major life-threatening intrathoracic injuries. Treatment for these precluded early spinal fixation and a fixed spinal deformity occurred without neurological injury.

THORACOLUMBAR INJURIES

The thoracolumbar region (T11–L2) is a high stress area of the spinal column, where the relatively stiff thoracic spine joins the more flexible lumbar spine. Mining accidents involving acute flexion and rotation injuries caused by rock falls provided most of the early examples of this injury. Nowadays, high-velocity road traffic accidents and falls from a height (horse riding, parachuting, gliding, and suicide attempts) account for the majority of cases.

Most thoracolumbar injuries are unstable and result in narrowing of the spinal canal. At this level the spinal canal may contain cord, cauda equina, or a combination of both. Identical bony injuries can result in a range of neurological lesions, varying from complete paraplegia to no deficit. Partial neurological lesions can be expected to have some recovery, particulary after surgical decompression and stabilization.

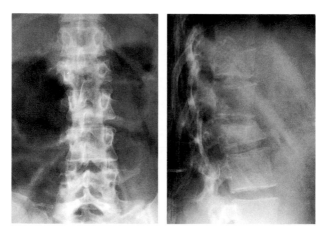

Fig.99 Radiographs of the spine following a suicide attempt. The patient jumped from a five storey building, sustaining a burst fracture of L1 with minimal disruption (left). The lateral view (right) indicates a normal contour of the posterior surface of the body of the vertebra, but the posterior body height is reduced and this suggests that a posterior burst fragment may be present.

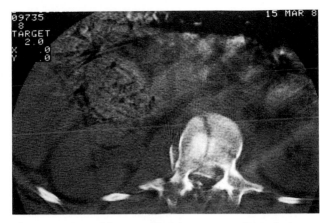

Fig.100 A CT scan of the same patient shows a more extensive fracture than initially suggested by the plain films. There is a large retropulsed fragment of bone from the intermediate column which is intruding into the spinal canal. Prior to CT scanning this type of injury was considered to be stable, but fractures through all three columns of the spine confirm that this is an unstable injury, and in this case, the patient sustained a severe cauda equina lesion.

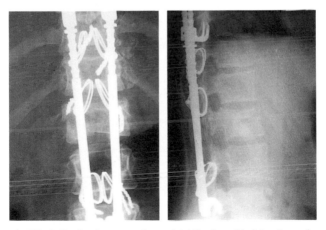

Fig.101 Following decompression and stabilization with distraction rods and sublaminar wires, the fracture was reduced and the patient made a full neurological recovery. The vertebral body was reconstituted, with restoration of body height.

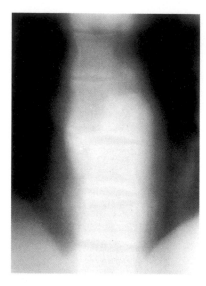

Fig.102 This shear fracture is shown by tomography, and usually results in paraplegia.

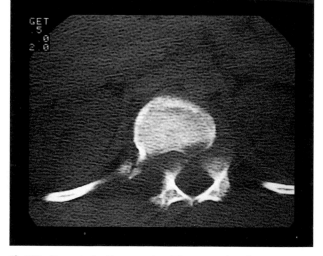

Fig.103 Computerized tomography of the same patient demonstrates a fracture through the base of both pedicles. Although the anterior column is intact, this fracture is unstable as the posterior column, and thus the ring, of the spinal cord is disrupted in two places. There was, surprisingly perhaps, no neurological deficit as the posterior column and spinal cord are not disrupted.

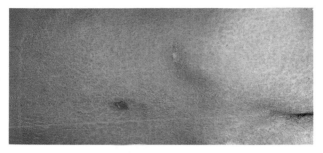

Fig.104 Careful examination of the torso usually reveals external evidence of underlying spinal injury. This minor contusion overlay a painful palpable irregularity of the spinous processes.

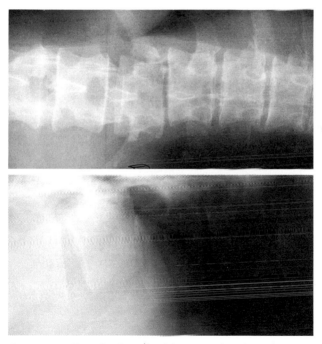

Fig.105 AP and lateral radiographs of the same patient show a fracture dislocation of T11–12 with less than 20% subluxation and no neurological deficit.

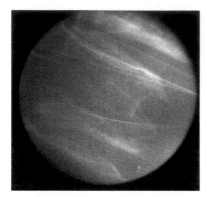

Fig.106 A Chance fracture is caused by a hyperflexion injury which involves bone only, with a transverse fracture through the vertebral body.

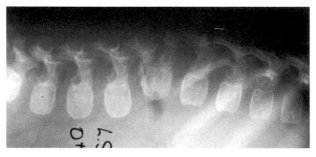

Fig.107 Although spinal injuries are uncommon in young children, they can occur in high velocity injuries. This highly unstable Chance fracture occurred in a 9-month-old baby. The injury was sustained during hyperflexion across a safety belt worn by the child's mother. The car in which they were travelling was involved in a head-on collision.

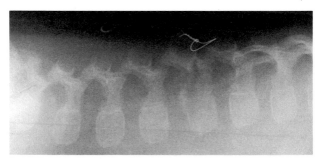

Fig.108 The spine was stabilized with a posterior wire but no recovery of a complete paraplegia occurred.

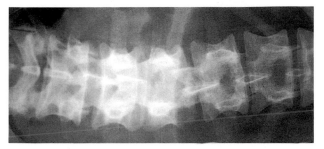

Fig.109 Unlike the cervical spine, where locked facets may occur owing to the horizontal orientation of the joints, locked facets in the lumbar spine, where the joints are vertical, is unusual.

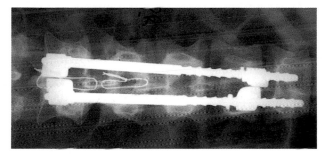

Fig.110 This example of a locked L1 – L2 facet was reduced and stabilized with Harrington rods.

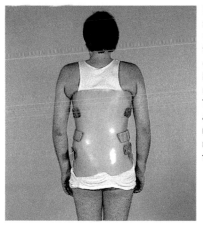

Fig.111 Following spinal stabilization, all patients are mobilized within a few days of surgery in a custom-made supportive body jacket, which can be removed for washing. The jacket is worn for approximately nine months, when rods are removed after healing of the fracture.

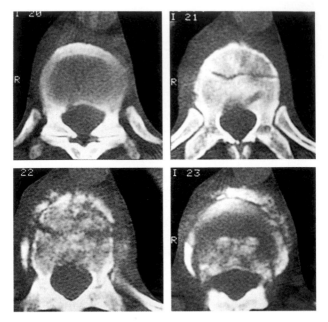

Fig.112 Posterior stabilization of late-presenting spinal injuries is futile, since the fracture is soon irreducible owing to fracture healing and callus formation, as seen in this CT scan of a burst fracture, taken 6 weeks after injury.

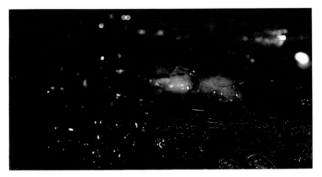

Fig.113 Anterior decompression and bone grafting is indicated if there is a partial or progressive neurological lesion with narrowing of the spinal canal. In this example, the vertebral body has been removed, the spinal canal decompressed and bone strut grafts inserted to support the anterior column of the spine.

THE LUMBAR SPINE

The Intervertebral Disc

Although bony injury is relatively uncommon in the lumbar spine, disc prolapse and other soft tissue injury to this region accounts for a great deal of spinal morbidity.

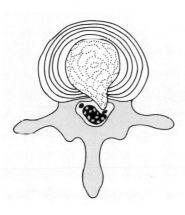

Fig.114 Minor twisting injuries may be sufficient to cause prolapse of an already degenerate nucleus pulposus of a lumbar disc through the anulus fibrosus. This example shows a posterolateral disc prolapse causing nerve root decompression.

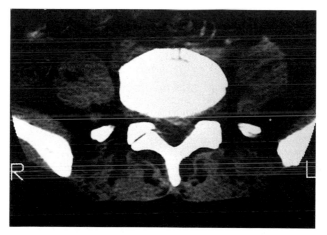

Fig.115 The midline is strengthened posteriorly by the posterior longitudinal ligament so the disc material rarely prolapses posteriorly but most commonly posterolaterally with compression of the nerve root as it enters the nerve root canal as seen in this CT scan.

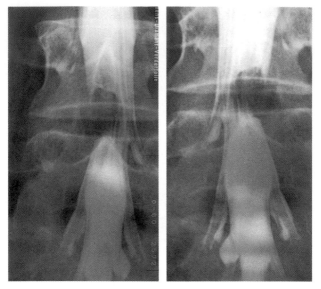

Fig.116 A myelogram showing a constant posterolateral filling defect at the L4–L5 disc level. The disc space is narrowed, suggesting that disc degeneration is long-standing.

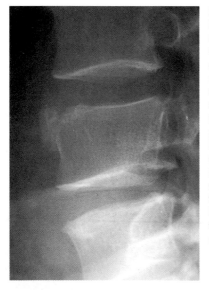

Fig.117 Minor bony injury may result in mild degrees of instability, with development of osteophytes and narrowing of the spinal canal. This man suffered a minimally displaced fracture of the upper end plate of L4, and 18 years later developed spinal stenosis owing to intrusion into the spinal canal of an osteophyte at the lower border of the body of L4. Removal of the bony fragment relieved his symptoms.

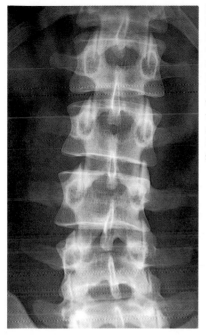

Fig.118 Fracture of lumbar transverse processes is caused by either direct injury or avulsion by strong paravertebral muscles (particularly psoas). As well as the fractures, plain films of the lumbar spine also show a scoliosis and loss of the normal psoas shadow.

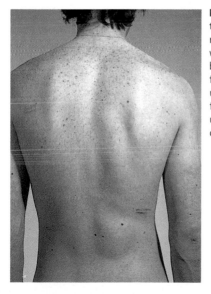

Fig.119 Examination of the back invariably reveals the scoliosis, as well as a swelling caused by muscle spasm and fracture haematoma. The urine should be checked for blood, as kidney or ureteric damage may occur with this injury.

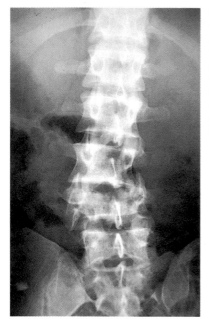

Fig.120 Burst fractures of the lumbar spine are often extensive and are usually caused by falls from a height. The extent of the injury may be obvious on a plain film, where separation of the pedicles indicates total disruption.

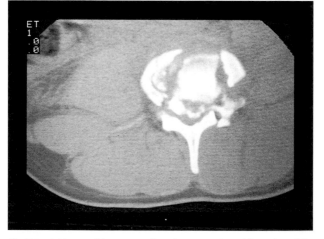

Fig.121 A CT scan of the same patient shows complete obliteration of the spinal canal. Perhaps surprisingly, such extensive bony damage rarely results in a complete lesion, as the cauda equina below L1 in the lumbar spine is much more resistant to permanent damage than the spinal cord.

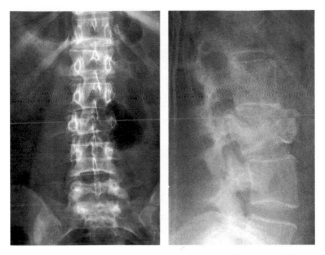

Fig.122 The lumbar spine of a young woman who fell from a roof. The AP view (left) shows obliteration of the left psoas shadow, with preservation of the right side. A loop of bowel gas overlies a burst fracture of L3. The lateral view (right) shows that fracture fragments of the body appear to protrude anteriorly more than posteriorly.

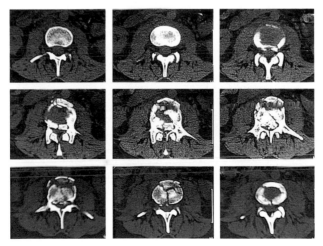

Fig.123 As is often the case, plain films are misleading and serial CT scans indicate the extent of the injury. In this case, the spinal canal has been obliterated by fragments of bone retropulsed from the body.

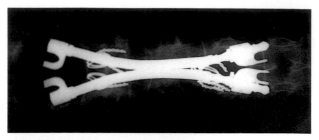

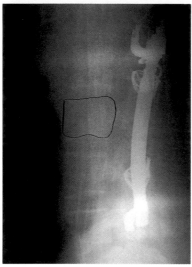

Fig.124 Laminectomy and stabilization with Harrington rods and sublaminar wires resulted in decompression of the spinal canal and restoration of the anatomy, with improvement of an incomplete neurological injury.

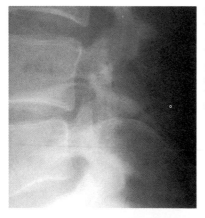

Fig.125 A direct blow to the midline lumbar region may cause a fracture of a spinous process. Such a fracture is stable and the only treatment needed is symptomatic.

Spondylolisthesis

Spondylolisthesis occurs most commonly in the lower lumbar region and is classified into the following categories:

- Spondylolytic
- Degenerative
- Pathological
- Congenital
- Traumatic

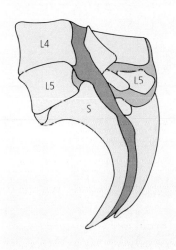

Fig.126 The essential feature of spondylolisthesis is discontinuity in the pars interarticularis, allowing the vertebral column to slip forward at the level of the lesion.

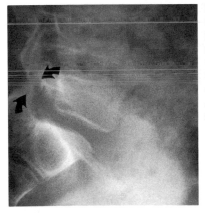

Fig.127 The commonest type of spondylolisthesis, is spondylolytic which is a stress fracture through the pars interarticularis. It is most commonly seen in children and young adults, and may cause symptoms in later life.

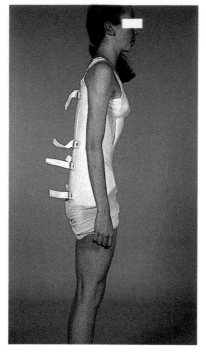

Fig.128 With early diagnosis and support in a brace, the fracture may heal. Symptomatic, progressive slipping requires spinal fusion.

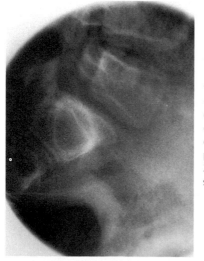

Fig.129 Traumatic spondylolisthesis is rare and requires extensive shearing forces to fracture both partes interarticulares. The fracture is usually complicated by disc disruption into the spinal canal. In this case, a wide defect is present at the pars interarticularis with a 25% slip of L5 on the sacrum.

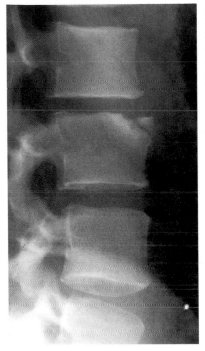

Fig.130 Changes resembling those of Scheuermann's disease can occur in the lumbar spine and may affect only one vertebral end plate. This 25-year-old man presented with back pain but no previous injury. Although only one vertebra is affected, anterior end plate irregularity with slight loss of disc height is characteristic of Scheuermann's disease.

INDEX